MENTAL HEALTH OF
ELDERLY STAYING IN OLD AGE HOMES

RAJ KUMARI VERMA

D1664411

Contents

CHAPTER 1

INTRODUCTION

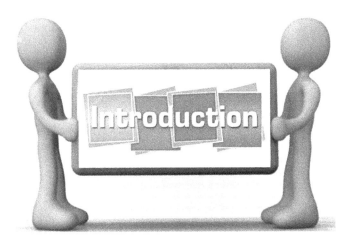

Long life is a sign of good health; and aging is a natural process that influences the individual, family and society in different ways. Ageing is not disease but the final stage of normal life. The ageing of the world's population in developing and developed countries is an indicator of improving global health. Since the beginning of century, the number of people over 65 years of age has increased worldwide. The age composition of the population of India has been undergoing change; there has been a progressive increase in both the number of persons aged by 60 years or over was 12 million of this 5.5 million were male & 6.6 million were female.(Saran S.2008)

Ageing is a normal progressive process, beginning at conception and ending in death. Ageing is not synonymous with diseases but diseases become more common as age progresses. Usually the diseases present with non-specific multiple symptoms that involve many organs1. Increasing age in the elderly is associated with the higher morbidity and frequent use of health services2. Their illness tends to be chronic with no simple cure. This makes them more dependent on the family, society and health services. (Mohdaznanmd, Aris samsul Draman 2007)

Life expectancy for the elderly in developed and developing countries has increased as a result of improvement in public health and medical advances , and the increase in the absolute and relative numbers of elderly people is one of the major features of the world demographic transition (Gupta &Sankar, 2003; Beaglehole& Bonita,2004). Just now sixty percent of the elderly people live in developing countries (Yang et. al.2011). Due to the increased longevity and life expectancy, the quality of life has been considered as an important issue, attracting the attention of the researchers working on aging (Hall et al., 2011).

When the World Health Organization (WHO) defined health as ‗a state of complete physical, mental and social well-being, not merely the absence of disease or infirmity'', it implied that the assessment of health and healthcare should not only include traditional measures of morbidity and mortality, but should also include a broader assessment of the Quality of life (Saxena et al., 2001; Saxena et al., 2002).

With attention to these facts, Quality of life is a critical consideration in national and international healthcare policies and decisions in each country. If health policies cannot provide attempts to add peace and mental and physical health to human generation, the advances in this regard are considered to be ineffective and perilous (Fahey et al., 2003).

On the other hand it has been demonstrated that people face different physiological and mental problems as a result of aging that have negative effects on their Quality of life (Do¨nmez & Gokkoca, 2005; Schwarz et al., 2007; Williams et al., 2009).

Age is an important determinant of mental illness. The overall prevalence of mental and behavioral disorders tends to increase with age due to the normal ageing of the brain, deteriorating physical health and cerebral pathology. Lack of family support and restricted personal autonomy are other important contributing factors. Psychiatric morbidity among elderly people is frequent, severe and diverse.

Disorders such as depression, anxiety, cognitive and psychotic disorders have a high prevalence in this segment of the population.

Studies show that up to 20% being cared for in the community and about 37% being cared for at the primary level are suffering from depression. The Indian aged population is currently the second largest in the world and is projected to rise from 70 million, according to the National Census of 2001, to almost 324 million by the year 2050, with serious social, economic and public health consequences. Global trends in the incidence and prevalence of geropsychiatric disorders are reflected in India too. (Dr. Anil Kumar 2011)

Aging is a universal human experience. It is multifaceted and incredibly diverse. This is capturing the world's attention as one of the major challenges of the present century. It represents one of the most profound social and economic challenges facing the globe and is likely to reshape the political, economic, and cultural agendas of the world.(Arunp2004)

According to Population Census 2011 there are nearly 104 million elderly persons (aged 60 years or above) in India; 53 million females and 51 million males. Both the share and size of elderly population is increasing over time. From 5.6% in 1961 the proportion has increased to 8.6% in 2011. For males it was marginally lower at 8.2%, while for females it was 9.0%. As regards rural and urban areas, 71% of elderly population resides in rural areas while 29 % is in urban areas. The sex ratio among elderly people was as high as 1028 in 1951, subsequently dropped and again reached up to 1033 in 2011. The life expectancy at birth during 2009-13 was 69.3 for females as against 65.8 years for males. At the age of 60 years average remaining length of life was found to be about 18 years (16.9 for males and 19.0 for females) and that at age70 was less than 12 years (10.9 for males and 12.3 for females).The old-age dependency ratio climbed from 10.9% in 1961 to 14.2% in 2011 for India as a whole. For females and males, the value of the ratio was 14.9% and 13.6% in 2011. In rural areas, 66% of elderly men and 28% of elderly women were working, while in urban areas only 46% of elderly men and about 11% of elderly women were working. The percent of literates among elderly persons increased from 27% in 1991 to 44% in 2011.The literacy rates among elderly females (28%) is less than half of the literacy rate among elderly males (59%). Prevalence of heart diseases among elderly population was much higher in urban areas than in rural parts.

The world scenario is that by 2025, the aged population is expected to increase more than 830 million. As per 1951 census, the population of elderly in India was 20 million as compared to 57 million in 1991, 77 million in 2001and it is projected to increase to 177 million by 2025. The number of elderly people would rise to about 324 million by the year 2050. In India, 3.8% population accounts for people above 65 years of age. It is expected that by 2030, elderly population will account for 21.8% of total population. Majority of the elderly are living in rural areas (57.35%) compared to urban areas which is 50.78%[2].

The graying of India has become more visible than ever in the urban area. People have become more materialistic and mechanical which has turned man away from man. Among families the elderly are left alone to fend for themselves. In the rural areas, elderly are considered as a financial burden on the family. These problems have paved way for the elderly to seek shelter in old age homes. As of now, not much importance has been given to geriatric care in India. The time has come to plan cost effective and community friendly approach for comprehensive health care delivery to the large geriatric population. (Kaur M.2011)

In homes, changing lifestyles, values of the newly married young people are posing problems of adjustment to the elderly. The effect of growing industrialization, urbanization and the consequent crunch on space has forced many elderly parents to lead a lonely life away from their home. A comparative study was done on elderly living in old age home and within family setup in Jammu. The result of the study revealed that most of the elderly felt the attitude of the younger generation is unsatisfactory towards them especially those who were in old age home.(Aruna et al.2010)

The ageing of population is an obvious consequence of the process of demographic transition. While the countries of the west have already experienced and have planned for their elderly population, it is only in the last one and half decades that countries in Asia too are facing a steady growth of the elderly, as a result of the decline in fertility and mortality, better medical and health care and improvements in the overall quality of life of people. (KaurM.2011)

Within Asia, as India and China are the two largest countries in the region, it is expected that they would have a significant proportion of the world's elderly because of their large population base. In fact, the situation in India presents two different scenarios with certain states grappling with curbing their high fertility rates while others, which have controlled high fertility rates, are already experiencing or are poised to experience an increase in their elderly population. (Kaur M.2011)

There has been a progressive increase in both the number and proportion of the aged in India over time, particularly after 1951. Between 1901 and 1951, the proportion of population over age 60 increased marginally from 5 percent to 5.4 percent, while by 2001 this had increased to 7.0 percent. When changes in the decadal growth rate in the general population are compared with those for the elderly population, it is noted that the latter grew at a relatively much faster rate than the general population, since 1951. Furthermore, the decadal percent increase in the elderly population for the period 2001-2011 is likely to be more than double the rate of increase of the general population.

The size of the elderly rose in absolute terms during the last century from 12 million in 1901 to approximately 71 million in 2001 and is likely to reach 113 million in 2016. Yet another feature of ageing in India is the fact that the proportion of elderly is much higher in the rural areas than in the urban areas. The sex-wise pattern of growth of elderly population reveals that the increase is greater among women in the recent past, which indicates that elderly women will outnumber elderly men in the future. (Directory of Old Age Homes in India, Help Age India, 2002).

There is therefore an urgent need to examine the various aspects of this new and fast growing population to ensure the design of appropriate policy and programs directed to meet the varied needs of this vulnerable and dependent group. India, like many traditional societies, today faces a unique situation in providing care for its elderly as the existing old-age support structures in the form of family, kith and kin, are fast eroding and the elderly are ill-equipped to cope alone with their lives in the face of infirmity and disability. The onus of caring for the elderly is therefore now much more on the state than the family and will necessitate the creation of adequate institutional support.

While the western countries have a fairly well organized network of institutions for the care of the elderly, the growth and development of these facilities in India, which began as early as 1901, still remains inadequate. As per recent statistic, there are 1018 old age homes in India today. Out of these, 427 homes are free of cost while 153 old age homes are on pay and stay basis, 146 homes have both free as well as pay and stay facilities and detailed information is not available for 292 homes. A total of 371 old age homes all over the country are available for the sick and 118 homes are exclusive for women. A majority of the old age homes are concentrated in the developed states including Gujarat (Directory of Old Age Homes in India, Help Age India, 2002

Old age is the age of mellow fruitfulness and ripeness. All the efforts of years start giving the desired fruit. One's childishness, immaturity and recklessness give place to maturity, sense of discretion and second judgment. It can be said that this is the age which is termed as a link between the past and the future which is still keeping alive the tradition and culture of a society or a community. Aged are the persons serving the family, society and nation by the experience and wisdom which they had gained throughout their life .

Old age or aging is more like a science. Scientifically aging is the deterioration of an organism resulting from the essentially irreversible changes intrinsic to all members of a species such that with the passage of time they become unable to cope with stresses of the environment thereby increasing the probability of death thus according to National Institute of Ageing – ―Ageing in human refers to multidimensional process of physical, psychological and social change." This biological change affects the individual's life style and may result in psycho–emotional problems (Ramamurti and Jamuna, 1999) but in our daily life, where attitudes, behavior, values, aesthetics rule matters there is more that can be defined as an old age. It is one experience that cannot be had otherwise. When the trails of experience and wisdom have made a lasting impression on the human himself, one can say he is never out of it. It is a gift which no one can refuse to take.

Every organism that is born must age with time and decay. So aging is a natural and universal process and no society or individual can escape it (Neuhaus and Neuhaus, 1982). It is a continuous process that begins with the conception and ends with the death. Old age is a part of aging which is associated with different conditions of changes occurring in one's life (Nair, 1993). It is very difficult to define old age. In Indian context people who have attained 60 years of age and above are considered old, where as in developed countries it begins only at 65 years, although the incapacities due to aging start much later i.e. in 70 – 75 years (Kapoor and Kapoor, 2001). The aged are also known as ―elderly", old people or senior citizens and are generally taken to be people above the age of 60. This age group is also known as ―geriatric age group". Due to dependence for personal requirements old age is sometimes called the ―second childhood" (Pankjam, 2005). But the transformations brought in our society sometimes make us scare of this stage as everyone of us has to face it one day.

In our Indian society old age is often regarded as a time when the vessel of life has become empty and a time when human development potentiality has come to an irreversible and inevitable halt. Old age is the greatest challenge that an individual is facing in the rapidly changing scenario although researches show that even late in life potential exists for physical, mental, and social growth and development. In view of life long experiences and wisdom elderly are precious resource not only for families but also for nation.

"As we begin the twenty first century, population ageing is poised to emerge as a pre-eminent worldwide phenomenon. The confluence of lowered fertility and improved health and longevity has generated growing numbers and proportions of older population throughout most of the world and India is not an exception." (An Ageing World: 2001). According to the Census 2001, the number of older persons in India was 70.6 million or 7.4%. Among the 7.4% of ageing population of India 60% population is still working means contributing to the economy (Mishra, et.al. 2003). It's not that the elders who do not participate in workforce do not contribute to the economy, only it is not taken into account. They contribute by bringing up grandchildren, doing voluntary service and often counsel and resolve conflict by virtue of their position which might not be possible if they continue working (The Hindu, 2004). That is why, for some, it is the golden period of life when they can live freely without job anxiety or it can be said that without setting alarm clock. Now they can spend more time with their spouse but this is the one side of coin as the other side of coin is quite shocking.

In ancient India old people were considered as guiding stars in Indian families since they were symbols of tradition, respect, wisdom and experience. They transmitted the values of tolerance, co-operation and concern for others as they had witnessed in their elders. Today the scenario has changed in terms of interrelationships and the family dynamics existing within the family which are the product of industrialization and urbanization. Industrialization, migration, urbanization and westernization have severely affected our value system (Anand, 2004).

In India elderly population depends heavily on family for economic and emotional support. The breaking of traditional social structure is going against the aged. In traditional family set up oldest man was the head of the family and administrator of the family property. The joint family structure, values and respect attached to aged provided emotional strength, security and adjustment to them but the gradual disappearance of joint families has contributed to the special problems of aged in our society which require different strategies of adjustment on their part. The problem of old age is attracting the attention of many social scientist and human development specialist. The declaration of 1982 and again in 1999as the international years for the aged and 1st October as aged people's day shows the seriousness of problem (Sundaram, 1999).

India is a country of villages with 80% people living in rural areas. (Bhatt, 2007) Modernization, urbanization, industrialization and other such processes have drastically affected the rural family structure in general. The fact of consumerism and individualistic attitude of youth has necessitated them to move away from villages to gain more comfort and achieve future goals in urban areas leaving behind the aged parents (Behura and Mohanty, 2005). In such situations the aged parents have to work and care for themselves unsupportedly.

Most of the families in rural areas are involved in farming which has no retirement age as such. People have to work for themselves as long as their health allows them. In this situation the elderly feel lonely and economically insecure and there by lead a life of uncertainty and tribulation resulting in depression, anxiety and dissatisfaction from life. (Kumar, 1999)

Bansal (2001) in her study on life style satisfaction of underprivileged old age couples in urban areas of Udaipur district and Saharan (2003) in her study on life style of aged couples of rural area of

Shri Ganganagar district found that the aged husbands and wives were satisfied with their life style. Saharan in her study reported that the aged residing in Ganganagar was physically fit active and comparatively leading a healthy life. Geographical variations may be one of the significant factors affecting the quality of life of people because of various regional, socio economic and climatic differences. In Udaipur district the climate is not being supportive from past 10 to 15 years for rural farming families. Due to this unfavourable climatic condition the rural youth is migrating towards the other parts of country and some of the elderly in agrarian families have to continue working in the field. In extended families, the married younger generation is usually reported to be less cooperative with the aged parents. Wherever there are extended families the younger generation have opted for a job and are not performing farming responsibilities. Such situations have an adverse effect on the elderly who feel economically insecure and stress prone. The male elderly are becoming alcoholic, regular smoker and tobacco chewer to avoid the stress they are facing in their life. Again these ill habits have adverse effect on their health, working abilities and familial and societal relationships with specific reference to their spouse. All these factors i.e. poor health of male elderly, absence of children's support and fulfillment of multiple responsibilities in the field as well as in the home may affect the expectations and satisfaction towards life of rural elder persons.

Hence there is a need to study the rural aged population so as to understand their life style in depth and their expectations from their society as they are the most precious experienced population of the country. Thus the present study was an effort to study the life style of rural aged couples, their expectations from self, family, and society, and the level of satisfaction in personal, familial and societal aspects.

The world's population is ageing rapidly. Between 2015 and 2050, the proportion of the world's older adults is estimated to almost double from about 12% to 22%. In absolute terms, this is an expected increase from 900 million to 2 billion people over the age of 60. Older people face special physical and mental health challenges which need to be recognized.

Over 20% of adults aged 60 and over suffer from a mental or neurological disorder (excluding headache disorders) and 6.6% of all disability (disability adjusted life years-DALYs) among over 60s is attributed to neurological and mental disorders. These disorders in the elderly population account for 17.4% of Years Lived with Disability (YLDs). The most common neuropsychiatric disorders in this age group are dementia and depression. Anxiety disorders affect 3.8% of the elderly population, substance use problems affect almost 1% and around a quarter of deaths from self-harm are among those aged 60 or above. Substance abuse problems among the elderly are often overlooked or misdiagnosed.

Mental health problems are under-identified by health-care professionals and older people themselves, and the stigma surrounding mental illness makes people reluctant to seek help.

Health problems old age people

Osteoporosis is one of the major health problems many old people face. Osteoporosis is a condition in which bones become very fragile. This will increase the chance of fracture due to decreased bone density. The risk for osteoporosis is more in women after menopause.

Macular Degeneration Vision deterioration is one of the most common health problems in old people. In macular degeneration, the macula, which helps to sense and transmit images to the brain, is affected. This medical condition is usually found in elderly people above the age of 50.

Hearing Loss Hearing loss is an important issue that many senior citizens face. The most common form of age-related hearing loss is presbycusis. Older people may need a hearing aid because the ability to hear high frequency sound may decrease over time.

Glaucoma is one among the health problems of old people, which is due to an increase in the fluid pressure inside the eye. This increased pressure will cause damage to the optic nerve resulting in loss of vision.

Alzheimer's disease Alzheimer's disease is another serious issue in the list of health problems of old age. Once you get Alzheimer's disease, your ability to remember and think will be affect Cognitive impairment will cause memory loss and your ability to correlate things and do calculations will decrease over time. The affected person will be confused and the ability to take up more than one task at a time will be affected.

Arthritis is a common condition that almost all old people have to face. This is mainly an autoimmune disease, which is characterized by joint pain and deformities. Arthritis commonly affects fingers, hips, knees, wrists, and spine.

Metabolic Syndrome Obesity and other related issues during old age are mainly due to metabolic syndrome. This may further lead to Type 2 diabetes, cardiovascular disease, cancer and high blood pressure. Emotional disturbance Health problems of old age are not limited to physical disabilities. Old age can affect your mental health also because of various social aspects. This may create discomfort both to you and your family. Make sure you discuss your problems with close of Old age can be a terrifying concept for many people. It is true that the regenerative capacity of the body will decline with old age, making you more prone to old age related health issues.

There are many studies going on about the various health problems of old age, which is called geriatrics. It is important to be prepared to face the various health issues that you may experience as you near your old age. Apart from physical health problems of old age, there will be mental stress and anxiety as well due to social reasons. Knowing the common health problems of old age people will help you manage your life and lifestyle to reduce its impact. Some planning and preparations can make your old age more beautiful. The ability to deal with health problems of old age will make the task easier. Here are some of the important health's problems of old age that you should know about. Awareness of these problems will help you to plan for an optimum health. Family and friend's that they can support you in every possible way.

Risk factors for mental health problems among older adults

Multiple social, psychological, and biological factors determine the level of mental health of a person at any point of time. As well as the typical life stress or common to all people, many older adults lose their ability to live independently because of limited mobility, chronic pain, frailty or other mental or physical problems, and require some form of long-term care. In addition, older people are more likely to experience events such as bereavement, a drop in socioeconomic status with retirement, or a disability. All of these factors can result in isolation, loss of independence, loneliness and psychological distress in older people.

Mental health has an impact on physical health and vice versa. For example, older adults with physical health conditions such as heart disease have higher rates of depression than those who are medically well. Conversely, untreated depression in an older person with heart disease can negatively affect the outcome of the physical disease.

Older adults are also vulnerable to elder abuse - including physical, sexual, psychological, emotional, financial and material abuse; abandonment; neglect; and serious losses of dignity and respect. Current evidence suggests that 1 in 10 older people experience elder abuse. Elder abuse can lead not only to physical injuries, but also to serious, sometimes long-lasting psychological consequences, including depression and anxiety.

Facility and services of old age homes

The Chavi shanti dhaam was established in the year 2005 at Jankipuram Lucknow. A home for guardian (elderly people) spread on 5000 sq. feet of area. The dhaam has been all facilities that are normally required for the person of old age. The well maintain extremely neat and clean premise provide the all important and much needed stimulating environment. They have been available facilities for meditation, yoga, and other suitable physical exercise. a common hall having suitable recreation facilities such as TV. News paper, magazines and games, besides a common prayer room for the followers of divers faiths and rich library. They were facilities the different section of room and give the different name for different rooms like. mamta chaya etc.

Aastha centre for geriatric medicine is uniquely qualified to provide both primary and specialty health care service for older adults. They have been facilities for checkups, vaccination; illness a specialist geriatric is ready all time. Other services included physical examination, comprehensive geriatric assessments, evaluation of memory loss and depression osteoporosis assessment evaluation of balance and falls continence and other concerns of older adults, nutrition counseling meditation evaluation, long term geriatric care skilled nursing geriatric Icu palliative care, cancer therapy.

Old age home (Apna Ghar) the organization is functioning women old age home with the residential capacity of 100 women at 106 Aadresh Vihar Kanchana Bihar Marg Adil Nagar Jagrani hospital ring road Lucknow for last 3year with the help of department of women welfare government of u.p.it is running in a huge building where all necessary accommodation for olds are easily available for meeting out there general requirement. It provides free facilities for food, cloth, medical facilities and recreational them, physician yoga teacher, counselor, nurse, cook, sanitation worker, watchman etc. The line department of state government is helping us to reach the old women. At present more than 65 old women who are orphan, homeless and socially discarded.

Sevarth Vriddha Aasham establish in 1993 Rajajipuram in Lucknow. A home for the person is spread on 2500 sq feet. Severth Vriddha Aashram are facility free of the ageing people they also available facilities food, music system. Worship place available, medical facilities, care giver facilities, security, drinking water supply by Jal Nigam.

Samarpan Old age home was established in the year 2005.It has 19 double bedrooms with attach bathroom. It also has two dormitory one for men with 8 bed and second for ladies. It has also yoga room, kitchen, dining hall, medical room, library, television, news paper, drinking water etc.

Various Policies and Programmes of Central Government for Elderly People

Several initiative steps for various policies and programs for the elderly have been taken by the government. Some of them have been discussed as below:-

National Policy for Older Persons (NPOP) 1999

The National Policy on older Persons was announced by the Central Government of India in the year, 1999 to reaffirm the commitment to ensure the well-being of the older persons. It was a step to promote the health, safety, social security and well-being of elderly in India. The policy recognizes a person aged 60 years and above as elderly. This policy enables and supports voluntary and nongovernmental

Organizations to supplement the care provided by the family and provide care and protection to vulnerable elderly people. It was a step in the right direction in pursuance of the UN General Assembly Resolution 47/5 to observe 1999 as International Year of Older Persons and in keeping with the assurances to elderly people contained in the Constitution. The policy envisages state support in a number of areas – financial and food security, healthcare and nutrition, shelter, education, welfare, protection of life and property etc. for the well being of elderly people in the country. The primary objectives of this policy are to:-

❖ Ensure the well-being of the elderly so that they do not become marginalized, unprotected or ignored on any count.

❖ Encourage families to take care of their older family members by adopting mechanisms for improving inter generational ties so as to make the elderly a part and parcel of families.

❖ Encourage individuals to make adequate provision for their own as well as their spouse's old age.

❖ Provide protection on various grounds like financial security, health care, shelter and welfare, including protection against abuse and exploitation.

❖ Enable and support voluntary and non-governmental organizations to supplement the care provided by the family and recognizing the need for expansion of social and community services with universal accessibility.

❖ Provide care and protection to the vulnerable elderly people by ensuring for the elderly an equitable share in the benefits of development.

❖ Provide adequate healthcare facility to the elderly.

❖ Promote research and training facilities to train care givers and organizers of services for the elderly.

❖ Create awareness regarding elderly persons to help them lead productive and independent life.

This policy has resulted in the opening of new schemes such as –

❖ Promotion of the concept of healthy ageing.

❖ Setting up of Directorates of Older Persons in the States.

❖ Training and orientation to medical and paramedical personnel in health care of the elderly. Assistance to societies for production and distribution of material on elderly care.

❖ Strengthening of primary health care system to enable it to meet the health care needs of older persons.

❖ Provision of separate queues and reservation of beds for elderly patients in hospitals.

❖ Extended coverage under the Antodaya Schemes especially emphasis for elderly people.

National Council for Older Persons (NCOP)

A National Council for Older Persons (NCOP) was constituted in 1999 under the chairpersonship of the Ministry of Social Justice and Empowerment to operationalize the National Policy on Older Persons. The NCOP is the highest body to advise the Government in the formulation and implementation of policy and programmes for the elderly. The basic objectives of this council are to:-

❖ Advise the Government on policies and programmes for older persons.

❖ Represent the collective opinion of elderly persons to the government.

❖ Suggest steps to make old age productive and interesting.

❖ Provide feedback to the government on the implementation of the

NCOP as well as on specific programmed initiatives for elderly.

❖ Suggest measures to enhance the quality of inter-generational relationships.

❖ Provide a nodal point at the national level for redressing the grievances of older persons which are of an individual nature provide lobby for concessions, rebates and discounts for older persons both with the Government as well as with the corporate sector.

❖ Work as a nodal point at the national level for redressing the grievances of elderly people. Undertake any other work or activity in the best interest of elderly people.

The council was re-constituted in 2005 and met at least once every year. At present there are 50 members in it, comprising representatives of Central and State Governments, NGO's, citizens' group, retired persons' associations, and experts in the fields of law, social welfare and medicine.

Central Sector Scheme of Integrated Programme for Older Persons (IPOP)

An integrated Programme for Older Persons (IPOP) is being implemented since 1992 with the objective of improving the quality of life of senior citizens by providing basic amenities like food, shelter, medical care and entertainment opportunities and by encouraging productive and active ageing. Under this scheme financial assistance up to 90 percent of the project cost is provided to Non-Governmental Organizations for running and maintenance of old age homes, day care centers and mobile medicine units. The scheme has been made flexible so as to meet the diverse needs of the older persons including reinforcement and strengthening of the family, awareness generation on issues pertaining to older persons, popularization of the concept of lifelong preparation for old age etc. Several innovative projects have also been added which are as follows:-

❖ Maintenance of respite care homes and continuous care homes.

❖ Sensitizing programmes for children particularly in schools and colleges.

❖ Regional resource and training centers for caregivers of elderly persons.

❖ Volunteer Bureau for elderly persons

❖ Formation of associations for elderly.

❖ Helplines and counselling centers for older persons.

❖ Awareness Generation Programmes for elderly people and caregiver.

❖ Running of day care centers for patients of Alzheimer's Disease/Dementia, and physiotherapy clinics for elderly people.

❖ Providing disability and hearing aids for the elderly people.

The eligibility criteria for beneficiaries of some important projects Supported under IPOP Scheme are:-

❖ Old age homes – for destitute elderly persons.

❖ Respite care homes and continuous care homes – for elderly persons who are seriously ill and require continuous nursing care and respite

❖ Mobile Medicare units – for older persons living in slums, rural and inaccessible areas where proper health facilities are not available.

The scheme has been revised in April, 2008. Besides an increase in amount of financial assistance for existing projects, Governments/ Panchayati Raj institutions/local bodies have been made eligible for getting financial assistance.

Inter-Ministerial Committee on Older Persons

An Inter-Ministerial Committee on Older Persons comprising twenty-two Ministries/Departments, and headed by the secretary, Ministry of Social Justice and Empowerment is another coordination mechanism in implementation of the NPOP. Action Plan on ageing issues for implementation by various Ministries/Departments concerned is considered from time to time by the committee.

National Old Age Pension (NOAP) Scheme

Under NOAP Scheme, in 1994 Central Assistance was available. The amount of old age pension varies in the different States as per their share to this scheme. It is implemented in the State and Union Territories through Panchayats and Minicipalities. The assistance was available on fulfillment of the following criteria:-

❖ 65 years or more should be the age of the applicant (male or female)

❖ The applicants who have no regular means of subsistence from their own source of income or through financial support from family members or others.

The Ministry is now implementing the Indira Gandhi National Old Age Pension Scheme (IGNOAPS). Under this scheme Central assistance in form of Pension is given to persons, above 65 years .Rs. 200/- per month, belonging to a below poverty line family. This pension amount is meant to be supplemented by at least same contribution by the States so that each applicant gets at least Rs. 400/- per month as pension. The number of beneficiaries receiving central assistance, in the form of pension, was 171 lakh as on 31st March, 2011.

Further the Ministry has lowered the age limit from the existing 65 years to 60 years and the pension amount for elderly of 80 years and above has also been increased from Rs. 200/- to Rs. 500/- per month with effect from 01.04.2011. This decision of the Government of India has been issued to all States/UTs vide letter no. J-11015/1/2011-NSAP dated 30th June, 2011.

National Programme for Health Care of Elderly (NPHCE)

National Programme for Health Care of Elderly (NPHCE) is an articulation of the international and national commitments of the government as envisaged under (UNCRPD), National Policy on older Persons (NPOP) adopted by the Government of India in 1999 and Section 20 of ―The Maintenance and Welfare of Parents and Senior Citizens Act, 2007" dealing with provisional for medical care of senior citizen. Ministry of Health and Family Welfare (MOHFW) has taken appropriate steps in this regard by launching the National Programme for Health Care of Elderly (NPHCE) as a centrally sponsored scheme under the new initiatives in the XI five years plan. Presently, it is being rolled out in 100 districts. The vision of the NPHCE is:

❖ To provide accessible, affordable and high quality long-terms comprehensive and dedicated care services to an Ageing population.

❖ Creating a new ‑architecture" for Ageing.

❖ To build a frame-work to create an enabling environment for ‑a society for all ages".

❖ To promote the concept of Active and Healthy Ageing.

❖ Convergence with National Rural Health Mission, AYUSH and other line departments like Ministry of Social Justice and Empowerment.

Specific Objectives of NPHCE are:

❖ To identify the health problems in the elderly and provide appropriate health interventions in the community with a strong referral backup support.

❖ To provide an easy access to promotional, preventive, curative and rehabilitative services to the elderly through community based primary health care approach.

❖ To build capacity of the medical and paramedical professional as well as the care-takers within the family for providing health care to the elderly.

❖ To provide referral services to the elderly patients through district hospitals, regional medical institutions. Core Strategies to achieve the objective of the Programme.

❖ Community based Primary Health Care approach including domiciliary visits by trained health care workers.

❖   Dedicated services at PHC/CHC level including provision of machinery, equipment, training, additional human resources (CHC), IEC etc.

❖   Dedicated facilities at District Hospital with 10 bedded wards, additional human resources, machinery, and equipment, consumable and drugs, training and IEC.

❖   Strengthening of 8 Regional Medical Institutes to provide dedicated tertiary level medical facilities for the elderly, introducing PG courses in Geriatric Medicine, and in-service training of health personnel at all levels.

❖   Information, Education and Communication (IEC) using mass media, folk media and other communication channels to reach out to the target community.

❖   Continuous monitoring and independent evaluation of the programme and research in Geriatrics and implementation of NPHCE. Promotion of public and private partnerships in Geriatric Health Care.

❖   Mainstreaming AYUSH – revitalizing local health traditions, and convergence with programmes of Ministry of Social Justice and Empowerment in the field of geriatrics.

❖   Reorienting medical education to support geriatric issues.

National Policy on Senior Citizens 2011

The foundation of National Policy for Senior Citizens 2011 is based on several factors – demographic explosion among the elderly, the changing economy and social milieu, advancement in medical research, science and technology and high levels of destitution among the elderly rural poor. In principle the policy values an age integrated society. It believes in the development of a formal and informal social support system, so that the capacity of the family to take care of senior citizens is strengthened and they continue to live in the family. All those of 60 years and above are senior citizens. This policy advocates issues related to senior citizens living in urban and rural areas, special needs of the _oldest old' and older women. It will endeavour to strengthen integration between generations, facilitate interaction between the old and the young as well as strengthen bonds between different age groups. It believes in the development of a formal and informal social support system, so that the capacity to the family to take care of senior citizens is strengthened and they continue to live in the family. The policy seeks to reach out in particular to the bulk of senior citizens living in rural areas who are dependent on family bonds and intergenerational understanding and support. The focus of the new policy:

❖ Promote the concept of _Ageing in Place' or ageing in own home, housing, income security and homecare services, old age pension and access to healthcare insurance schemes and other programmes and services to facilitate and sustain dignity in old age. The thrust of the policy would be preventive rather than cure.

❖ Mainstream senior citizens, especially older women, and bring their concerns into the national development debate with priority to implement mechanisms already set by governments and supported by civil society and senior citizens' associations. Support promotion and establishment of senior citizens' association, especially amongst women.

❖ The policy will consider institutional care as the last resort. It recognizes that care of senior citizens institutional care as the last resort. It recognizes that care of senior citizens has to remain vested in the family which would partner the community, government and the private sector.

❖ Long term savings instruments and credit activities will be promoted to reach both rural and urban areas. It will be necessary for the contributors to feel assured that the payments at the end of the stipulated period are attractive enough to take care of the likely erosion in purchasing power.

❖ Being a signatory to the Madrid Plan of Action and Barrier Free Framework it will work towards an inclusive, barrier-free and age friendly society.

❖ Recognize the senior citizens are a valuable resource for the country and create an environment that provides them with equal opportunities, protects their rights and enables their full participation in society. Towards achievement of this directive, the policy visualizes that the states will extend their support for senior citizens, living below the poverty line in urban and rural areas and ensures their social security, healthcare, shelter and welfare. It will protect them from abuse and exploitation so that the quality of their lives improves.

❖ Employment in income generating activities after superannuation will be encouraged.

❖ States will be advised to implement the Maintenance and Welfare of Parents and Senior Citizens Act, 2007 and set up Tribunals so that elderly parents unable to maintain themselves are not abandoned and neglected.

❖ Support and assist organizations that provide counseling, career guidance and training services.

❖ States will set up homes with assisted living facilities for abandoned senior citizens in every district of the country and there will be adequate budgetary support.

SOME OTHER IMPORTANT ACTIVITIES

Some of other important activities regarding the welfare of elderly people are as follows:-

International Day of Older Persons

The International Day of Older Persons is celebrated every year on 1st October, 2009. On 01.10.2009, the Hon'ble Minister of Social Justice and Empowerment flagged off ―Walkathon" at Rajpath, India Gate, to promote inter-generational bonding. More than 3000 senior citizens/elderly people from across Delhi, NGOs working in the field of elderly issues, and school children from different schools participated in this.

❖ The government has launched various scheme and policies for elderly have been taken by the voluntary agencies in India. Provide feedback to the government on the implementation of the scheme.

❖ Improving their situation through government and nongovernment efforts in providing relief measures for economic assistance, health care and legal awareness services. Measure the success would be elimination of policy.

❖ Monitoring and evaluation would be needed to ensure equitable outcomes for older people.

CHAPTER 2

REVIEW OF LITERATURE

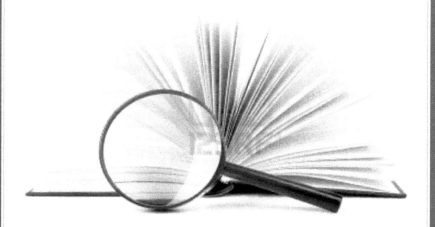

This chapter presents the literature relevant to the topic. An overall research calls for a clear perception in the field of study and proves to be helpful for the execution of a research study in order to provide clear and better understanding the literature reviewed for the present study. Review of literature refers to an extensive, exhaustive and systematic examination of population relevant t the study. It is an essential part of every research, which helps to support the hypothesis under the study and to critically analyze the structure and content of the research report. A comprehensive review is mandatory in any research endeavor. This require thorough efforts on the part of the investigator to select relevant subject matter, to select organize and to report it systematically. An in depth literature review facilitates in knowing the trend of thought and research already done in specific area of work. This chapter deals with brief account of literature, which has direct and indirect bearing on the specific objectives of the investigation.

> ➤ Aging and its concepts
> ➤ Function and services of old age home
> ➤ Mental health of elderly
> ➤ Health problem of elderly
> ➤ Various problems in smooth functions of old age homes

"Trees grow stronger over the years, rivers wider. Likewise, with age, human beings gain immeasurable depth and breadth of experience and wisdom. That is why older persons should not only be respected and revered; they should be utilized as the rich resource to society that they are" (Annan. 2003)

Ageing is a natural process that begins at birth, or to be more precise, at conception, a process that progresses throughout one's life and ends at death. (Hernandez, 2002). Ageing is a constant, predictable process that involves growth and development of living organisms. Aging can't be avoided, but how fast one ages varies from one person to another. How, one ages depends upon the genes, environmental influences, and life style (Smith, 2004). Ageing can also be defined as a state of mind, which does not always keep pace with the chronological age. Attitude and how well an individual face the normal changes, challenges and opportunities of later life may best define the age (Arber, 2004).

(Tiwari 1999) defined as a decline in physiological competency that increases the incidence and intensities of vulnerability to accidents, diseases and other form of environment stresses. Swarnlata (2000) Comments that along with a generalized decrease in body's physiological efficiency, the social adjustment of elderly people also gets affected. Bhatt (2007) adds that the physical and social changes are accompanied by psychological changes in the elderly. These changes have profound effect on personal and social adjustments on elderly people. Ageing refers to three groups of older adults: the young old, old –old and oldest old. Chronologically young old generally refers to people aged 65 to 74, who are usually active, vital and vigorous. The old -old, aged 75 to 84 and the oldest old aged 85 and above, are more likely to be frail and infirm and to have difficulty managing daily activities of daily living. (Papillae et.al, 2004)

Kapoor and Kapoor (2001) state that it is very difficult to define old age. In Indian context people who have attained 60 years of age and above are considered old, where as in developed countries it begins only at 65 years, although the incapacities due to aging start much later i.e. in 70 – 75 years.

The aged are also known as ―elderly", old people or senior citizens and are generally taken to be people above the age of 60. This age group is also known as ―geriatric age group". Due to dependence for personal requirement old age is sometimes called the ―second childhood" (Pankjam, 2005).

Population ageing is the most significant result of the process known as demographic transition. Reduction of fertility leads to a decline in the proportion of the young in the population. Reduction in the mortality means a longer life span for individuals. Population ageing involves a shift from high fertility/ mortality to low fertility / mortality and consequently increased proportion of older people in the total population. India is undergoing such a demographic transition. (Ghosh, 2001)

Ageing in India is a result of success in reducing fertility and mortality, this is a positive sign but what needs to be remembered is that ageing affects a whole range of issues. It has an effect on relationships within the family, more parents per child so to speak and finally an older generation, which will look to a younger generation to support it (Times of India, 27th April 2001).

As we begin the twenty first century, population ageing is poised to emerge as a pre-eminent worldwide phenomenon. The confluence of lowered fertility and improved health and longevity has generated growing numbers and proportions of older population throughout most of the world, while on one hand, population ageing represents a human success story, on the other, the steady, sustained growth of older people poses myriad challenges to policy makers and societies all over the world (kapoor, 2001).

The rising life expectancy at birth is one of the major achievements of the 20th century. But instead of rejoicing over the favourable demographic indicator, the world is caught in an "age-quake". For, the proportion of people aged 60 plus is rising and is expected to accelerate in the next 50 years. This "demographic time bomb" is nearing explosion in developed nations, and Asia including India is not far behind and this age quake is somewhat responsible for the status of elderly in the present society (Raghu, 2004)

Alphonsa K K et al. (2018) has conducted a study effectiveness of relaxation therapy on psychological variables among the elderly in old age homes-A pilot study embarks on the effect of relaxation therapy on the psychological problems of the elderly in old age homes. Twenty elderly in the age group of 60-80 of both genders were included in the study after voluntary informed constant. Relaxation therapy (Jocobson's progressive muscles relaxation with music physical exercise, are laughter therapy) was given for an hour each in the morning and evening for 4 month successfully. Finding the study, it is evident that alternative therapies are greatly useful in geriatric care and it could be recommended for the psychological health and well being of the elderly.

Eun-Hi Kong (2015) has conducted a study Agitation in dementia: concept clarification a transition from the observer's perspective to the patient's perspective in the interpretation of agitation was found. Five critical attributes of agitation in dementia were identified: excessive, inappropriate, repetitive, non-specific and observable. Patient factors, interpersonal factors, environmental factors and restraint were identified as precipitating antecedents. Mediating antecedents included discomfort, unmet need and misinterpretation. Consequences of agitation were identified at the levels of patient, caregiver and others.

Bjorkaf (2013) Has conducted a study coping and depression in old age seventy-five studies, 38 clinical and 37 community settings, were included. Of these, 44 were evaluated to be of higher quality. Studies recruiting samples of older persons with a major depressive disorder, moderate or severe cognitive impairment or those who were dependent on care were scarce, thus the research is not representative of such samples. We found a huge variety of instruments assessing resources and strategies of coping (55 inventories). Although we found the relation between resources and strategies of coping and depression to be strong in the majority of studies, i.e. a higher sense of control and internal locus of control, more active strategies and positive religious coping were significantly associated with fewer symptoms of depression both in longitudinal and cross-sectional studies in clinical and community settings. Resources and strategies of coping are significantly associated with depressive symptoms in late life, but more research to systematize the field of coping and to validate the instruments of resources and strategies of coping in older populations is required, especially among older persons suffering from major depression and cognitive decline.

J. Heydari, S. Khaniet al. (2012) has conducted a study life expectancy increases, the importance of elderly people's quality of life becomes more apparent.. The data are drawn from 220 elderly (>60 years of age) sampled from both settings. Data were analyzed using descriptive and inferential statistics. The average scores for several domains including total physical health, total mental health and overall health (total SF-36 score) were less than 50, which can be interpreted as a less desirable level of health-related quality of life in Iranian elderly people.. There is a need to design programs to increase elderly people's interaction with others and establish social networks for them and opined that these may enhance a sense of positive quality of life among the elderly.

S.C.Tiwari and Nisha M. Pandey (2012) has conducted a study improvements in health care services in India, the longevity and life expectancy have almost doubled. As a result, there is significant demographic transition, and the population of older adults in the country is growing rapidly. Epidemiological surveys have revealed enormous mental health morbidity in older adults (aged 60 years and above) and have necessitated immediate need for the development of mental health services in India. A differing, but in many aspects similar, picture emerged with regard to human resource and infrastructural requirements based on the two norms for the country to meet the challenges posed by psychiatrically ill older adults. A running commentary has been provided based on the available evidences and strategic options have been outlined to meet the requirements and minimize the gap. There is an urgent need to develop the subject and geriatric mental health care services in India.

Aruna Dubey and Seema Bhasin (2011) A study was conducted to understand the feeling of the elderly residing in the old age homes and within the family setup in Jammu. The sample of elderly women was selected using the ‑Purposive sampling" technique to select 30 elderly women from the old age home as well as a similar number from the family setups. Results of the study revealed that most of the elderly felt the attitude of the younger generation is unsatisfactory towards them especially those who were in old age homes in terms of getting respect, love and affection from the family members instead they were considered as burden for others. Women living in the families had a positive attitude towards old age.

Maria Cecilia et.al study conducted from 1980 to 2008. Fifty-two references were selected and analyzed. They showed a strong relationship among suicide ideation, attempt and completion in elderly individuals, which results from the interaction of complex physical, mental, neurobiological and social factors. Suicide associated with depression in the elderly can be prevented, provided the person is properly treated. In Brazil, it is necessary to invest in research, given the persistent increase in suicide rates among aged people, especially among males.

Saran S. (2009) study was conducted, among 32 residents of three skilled nursing homes to document the nature of the stressors they experienced and the coping mechanisms they used. The design used for this study was the one-shot case study. The sample comprised 26 (81%) women. Of the participants, 41% were 85 years or older, 31% were 75 to 84 years, and 28% were 74 years and younger. The findings indicated that medical issues were the most common stressors. The most common coping responses were prayer, reading, watching television, listening to music, and talking to friends and family.

Mathew M A (2009) has conducted a study in 2008 to assess the stress, coping strategies and quality of life of institutionalized and non-institutionalized elderly in Kottayam district, Kerala. Data used in this study were collected from an old age home and a village in Kottayam with sample of 150 respondents aged 60 or older The survey used different tools such as socio-demographic proforma for institutionalized and non-institutionalized elderly, stress rating scale, a coping inventory, and WHOQOL-BREF scale. The study reveals that institutionalized elderly have more stress and less quality of life compared to non-institutionalized ones.

Kavitha A K (2008) A study was conducted in 2007 to find out quality of life of 50 senior citizens living in home for aged and 50 senior citizens living in the family set up in Erode district. The findings indicated that majority of senior citizens in the home for aged had moderate quality of life. Over all mean score regarding quality of life was found higher among senior citizens living in family set up than the senior citizens living in home for the aged.

Sreevani R. (2007) A study was conducted in 2005 to assess the emotional problems among 50 elderly people in a selected old age home at Kolar District. Study revealed that most of the respondents (54 %) were between the age group of 60-70 years, 32% between 71-80 years and remaining (14%) above 80 years. Most of the respondents (68%) were male and 32% of them were females. Majority 80% of the subjects were suffering with major health problems. There was a association between sex and emotional problems of elderly people, there was significant association between emotional problems and general health status of elderly people.

Sreevani R. (2007) studies was done to assess the emotional problems among elderly people in a selected old age home at Kolar district. A sample of 50 elderly people was selected using purposive sampling technique. Major findings of the study revealed that most of the respondents (54%) were between age groups of 60-70yrs. Sixty eight percent of respondents were males and 32% of them were females. Majority of them were having minor emotional problems (54%) and the remaining (46%) were healthy. There was significant association between sex and emotional problems of elderly people.

Nisha N. (2007) has conducted a study emotional wellbeing of elderly staying in old age home versus elderly staying in the family. The major findings of the study was that, majority of the senior citizens (90%) from old age home had a borderline emotional wellbeing, 5% of them had positive emotional wellbeing and rest of them had a negative emotional wellbeing, whereas among senior citizens staying in the family, 92% of them had a positive emotional wellbeing and 0.8% had border line personality.

Kavitha M. S. (2007) A study was done to determine the quality of life among senior citizens living in home for the aged and family setup in Erode district. This study revealed that majority of the senior citizens living in old aged homes had moderate quality of life and senior citizens living in families reported high quality of life.

Chakrabathi D. (2007) in their study to assess the wellbeing of elderly residing in old age home versus those in family setting. The main objective of the study was to assess subjective well-being of the elderly living in old age homes and family settings, assess level of satisfaction of the elderly living in old age homes and family setup as well as to find the relationship between subjective wellbeing of the elderly and their level of satisfaction. The major findings of the study included mean difference of subjective wellbeing of elderly living in family setting was significantly higher than elderly living in old age homes.

Kaur and Gaur (2003) A comparative study was conducted to assess the life satisfaction of institutionalized and non-institutionalized elderly in Chandigarh. About 200 elderly (32 institutionalized and 168 non-institutionalized) over 60 years of age were interviewed using a standard scale. Result indicated that life satisfaction of non-institutionalized elderly were found to be higher compared to institutionalized elderly, non-institutionalized male had better life satisfaction than institutionalized male.

Sijuwade (2003) A study was conducted to examine the subjective wellbeing of Nigerian urban elderly. About 200 elderly aged 60 or older were interviewed in relation to their family structure and relations, living arrangements, daily activities, health problems and old age concern as well as demographic concern to compare the both in relation to their perception of wellbeing and satisfaction of later life. Result indicated that males were having more wellbeing than females and the most significant findings of the study was the association between income and subjective wellbeing which suggest that the respondents who were economically better off were more likely to have a greater sense of well-being. This study shows that life satisfaction and wellbeing of the Nigerian elderly were closely associated with changes in social and family structures.

Shawn U O et.al. (2002) A study was conducted in 2002 among 127 elderly African Americans for examining the relationship among race related stress, quality of life indicators and life satisfaction. The findings indicated that there was an overall statically significant result for the gender (F=7.14, P<0.001). Elderly African American men And Women differed significantly with regard to institutional racism related stress (F = 12.63,p<0.01).

Ann Z Swimmer, (2002) Decreasing strength is the general physical change in the elderly. The sociologic issues of ageing are concerned with work, retirement, social security , health care and the response to getting old age is related to lifelong habits ,diet and exercise patterns. Old aged often becomes anxious if they live alone, lacking family support, poor income, accommodation and insecurity which may lead to depression.

Rammurthi (2001) A study was conducted to assess quality of life of institutionalized elderly in Andhra Pradesh. About 647 elderly over 60 years were interviewed using a standardized questionnaire which included reason for joining old age homes, the level of satisfaction and general feelings regarding subjective quality of life evaluation of their relationship with staff of the institution and overall satisfaction with life at that moment. This study indicated the need for improving the quality of life of elderly in old age homes.

Rajan et. al., (2004) conducted a survey of elders in old age homes in Pondicherry to find out problem of the aged reveals that a sizeable majority of the aged suffer from loss of memory and no sleep. Psychologically maximum number of the aged feels isolated, frustrated and depressed.

Morris (2006) states that Depression causes confusion and exacerbates dementia. It reduces a person's incentive to care for him, and lowers his energy level. Untreated depression could cause irreversible brain damage and could lead to suicide. It is one of the most common emotional and psychological disorders found in the elderly and affects relational problems. Later life depression can have serious repercussions in increasing mortality and disability, health care utilization and longer hospital stays, yet 63% older adults with a mental health disorder experience an unmet need for mental health service. Deteriorating health, a sense of isolation and hopelessness and difficulty adjusting to new life leads to depression and which in turn leads to suicide.

Majumdar (2001) has expressed the increase in the elderly population and their specific needs and problems saw the emergence of varied welfare measures providing for the elderly. The existing services such as daycare centers, old age institutions, social work services, senior citizen associations, voluntary organizations and other services for the elderly have been discussed with suggestions to provide for the specific needs of the elderly. The pivotal role of the voluntary organization in the welfare of the elderly especially in promoting their familial and social integration across all sections of society 76 has been discussed in great detail. Keeping in view the need to enlarge and strengthen the services for the elderly, cooperation from the family, community, government, professionals, researchers and from the elderly themselves have been suggested.

Mehta and Shrinagarpur (2000) state that ageing is a normal inevitable and universal phenomenon. Ageing is a process, which is universally independent of environmental factors, progressive, irreversible and likely to reduce functional competence.

Kumar (1992) stated that ageing is a toil some treadmill grinding to a tragic halt as the years pile up. It is a life spanning process of growth and development running from birth to death. It is generally associated with decline in the functional capacity of the organs of the body due to physiological transformation. During the process of ageing, physical functions of the body slowly deteriorate demanding greater coping skills on the part of the ageing person to adjust to the environment. In addition, there are problems caused by others in the society because of their unfavourable attitudes. Ageism, like sexism or racism, is a concept pertaining to prejudice or a negative attitude towards a particular group. Ageism implies that the old are perceived as sick, unhappy, empty and useless, and are discriminated against (Brittanica, 2005)

As the number of old people have gone up, quality of life has gone down. Industrialization, migration, urbanization and westernization have severely affected value systems. The erstwhile joint family, the natural support system, has crumbled. The fast-changing pace of life has added to the woes of the older person. (Rajgopalachari, 2003)

But there are regional variations in terms of living conditions, availability of resources and facilities. In general aged living in rural areas have poor sanitary conditions and less access to education and health facilities (Naik, 2001)

Bhadra (2000) stated that as a person grows older he tries to withdraw himself from active himself from active roles in family and tries to concentrate on activities outside the home like religious activities and other social activities as he is not so much capable of taking decisions in family now. Lakshmy (2003) supported the study and revealed that as persons grows older there is decline in abilities to adjust with new roles as a result of which elderly becomes more religious and more socially active in this age as they are not able to accept the passive role in family.

(2007) in his study on life style and health of elderly found that a higher percentage of male elderly with low and higher standard of living consume alcohol and beat their wife and children because of various frustrations.

Pawar (2001) in his study on the grandparent-grandchildren relationship in rural areas of Maharashtra found that as the youth is migrating towards the urban areas the grandparents are raising their grandchildren alone and this might be the reason for finding good grandparent- grandchild relationship.

Chakravarty (2001) reveals the vulnerability of the poor elderly and those in the unorganized sector has been the focus of several studies in view of the inadequate social security measures which increases their risk of becoming social and economic burdens in old age. The single most significant form of social assistance to the elderly in the unorganized sector is the Old Age Pension (OAP) scheme. Empowering the female elderly by improving their situation through governmental and non-governmental efforts in providing relief measures for economic assistance, health care, legal awareness and assistance and change in the attitude of the family, society and service providers have been suggested by several researchers.

Goel and Garg (2002)Due to breakdown of joint family system and tremendous influence of modern life styles on younger generation, the attitude of young people towards old age is constantly changing. Old people in the house become a sort of burden and liability. It is rather difficult for elderly to change their views and opinions suddenly to adjust with younger generation and that is why the term generation gap is becoming so popular in families.

Pradeep Kumar (2012) showed more females than males and the largest age group was the old-old. In a survey of all old age homes in the state of Kerala, India 64% was females and 36% in old-old age group compared to 32% in young-old and 21% in oldest old group.13 Thus the age and gender structure of the sample can be assumed not to skewed. In the present study most of the males were educated (60%), financially independent (75%) and thus may be considered as having better socio-economic status. In contrast, majority of the females had poor socio-economic status as 32% of them were illiterate or just literate (12%), widow (88%) and financially dependent (84%).

Saharan (2003) life style, expectations and problems of rural aged couples of Sri Ganganagar dist found that aged were living a healthy life style with no health problems and maintaining a good relation with their spouse and children as they were consult before taking any occupational and familial decision. Their participation in societal activities was also found to be good.

Bansal (2001) in her study on ‒life style satisfaction of underprivileged aged couples" revealed that more than two third of the aged couples were involved in their personal, familial and societal activities and moderate involvement was found in familial matters.

Waldron (2003) reported that in Indian family structure mother is a strong supporter of her children and a greater interaction has been found between mother and child which leads to greater expectations from children regarding care and concern and specially care of her husband and father of her children but when these expectations are not fulfilled conflicts occur in their relation and especially with daughter in law.

Rammurti (2001) reported that in rural areas most of the elderly expect that their children will fulfil their basic needs. The expectations are reportedly high from male child than the female child.

Saharan (2003) in her study on expectations of rural aged couples of Sri Ganganagar dist. found that the level of expectations of aged couples from their family members was found to be moderate this was in view of their good health and sound economic condition. However the expectations were high for emotional support from family and social support from society.

Mroczek. (2005) in a study on 1,927 men in New Zealand found that life satisfaction changes with age but this change may vary from individual to individual.

Gimpson (2003) who reported that high socioeconomic group people do have superior satisfaction from life as compared to lower socioeconomic group.

Easterlin (2003) in a study revealed that to become partially or completely dependent on others in old age, the loss of independence with its perceived rejection by society is feared by most elderly which gradually affect their satisfaction with life. Further **Syckle (2006)** adds that physical dependence due to disease or accident and economic dependence are the main fears in the elderly.

Agrawal (2002) in a study found that life satisfaction in rural elderly is comparatively high in people having land for agriculture, good economic conditions and good familial and societal relations.

Devarakonda (2007) in his study on insecurities in rural elderly of Uttar Pradesh on a sample of 2758 elderly found that the gravest fear of elderly concern living alone, poor health and monetary problems. The reasons cited for insecurity are largely health problems, followed by shortage of money and finally living alone. Though physical insecurity is not as pronounced as economic and health insecurity.

Lena k Ashok et al (2009) study showed that a major proportion of the elderly were out of the work force, partially or totally dependent on others, and suffering from health problems with a sense of neglect by their family members. There is a growing need for interventions to ensure the health of this vulnerable group and to create a policy to meet the care and needs of the disabled elderly. Further research, especially qualitative research, is needed to explore the depth of the problems of the elderly.

Max *et al.* (2005) revealed that the presence of perceived loneliness contributed strongly to the effect of depression on mortality. Thus, in the oldest old, depression is associated with mortality only when feelings of loneliness are present. Depression is a problem that often accompanies loneliness. In many cases, depressive symptoms such as withdrawal, anxiety, lack of motivation and sadness mimic and mask the symptoms of loneliness.

Banerjee and Tyagi, (2003) Aging is a normal inevitable and universal phenomenon. Increase of aged population throughout the world has attracted the attention of social scientists. Apart from different factors, old age has many psychological manifestations. Due to generation gap, change of value system, breaking up of joint family etc. the ageing has become a complex and challenging proposition for the aged individual. The roles and status of aged have changed and the knowledge and experience of old people has lost significance in urban as well as in rural society. On the contrary, the aged people can not accept easily the prescribed role of their contemporary situation. This role conflict creates a kind of tension, maladjustment and dissatisfaction from life among the aged. Economic insecurity has also played a vital role in this regard.

Reddy subramaniyam G. (2005) stated that global population ageing is an important challenge and action has to be taken by virtually all countries .The geriatric population was about 600 million in 2000.It is expected to raise up to 1.2 billion in 2025 and 2 billion in 2050.About two thirds of all older persons are living in the developed countries this figure, by 2025 will be about 75%. In developing countries like India these figures have changed the nature of demands on the health care system. Health delivery system has to accommodate the needs of the older population.

White et al., (2006) conducted study on cognitive, emotional and quality of life outcomes in patients with pulmonary arterial hypertension. Results shows that cognitive sequelae occurred in 58 percent (27/46) of the pulmonary arterial hypertension patient's .Patients with cognitive sequelae had worse verbal learning delayed verbal memory, executive function, and fine motor scores compared to patients without cognitive sequelae. 26 percent of patients had moderate to severe depression and 19 percent had moderate to severe anxiety. Depression, anxiety and quality of life were not different for patients with or without sequelae. Patients had decrease quality of life, which was associated with worse working memory.

Andreoletti et. al., (2006) conducted a study on age differences in the relationship between anxiety and recall. The results shows that a negative relationship between cognitive-specific anxiety and memory, such that greater anxiety was related to poor recall, but this was so only for middle aged and older results suggest that managing anxiety may be a promising avenue for minimizing episodic memory problems in later life.

Routaslo et. al., (2006) study conducted on social contacts and their relationship to loneliness among aged people results declares that more than one third of the respondents39.4suffered from loneliness. Feeling of loneliness was not associated with the frequency of contacts with children and friends but rather with expectations and satisfaction of these contacts. The most powerful predictors of loneliness were living alone, depression, experienced poor understanding by the nearest and unfulfilled expectations of contacts with friends.

Rajan et. al., (2004) conducted a survey of elders in old age homes in Pondicherry to find out problem of the aged reveals that a sizeable majority of the aged suffer from loss of memory and no sleep. Psychologically maximum number of the aged feels isolated, frustrated and depressed.

Wilson K (2006)[1] conducted a study reveals that a prevalence rate of 21 percent and an annual incidence of 12.8 percent (Geriatric depression score of five or more) were found Risk factors associated with prevalence depression include not living close to friends and family ,poor satisfaction with living accommodation and poor satisfaction with finances.Subsequent development of clinically significant depressive symptoms was associated with base line increased scores in depression.

Sherina M. S et. al., (2006) the prevalence of depression among elderly in a tertiary care center in Wilayah Persekutan.The results showed that 54 percent of the elderly respondents were found to have depressive symptoms age ,sex, ethnicity, functional disabilities in bathing, grooming, dressing, using the toilet, transferring from bed to chair and back, mobility and climbing chairs were all found to be significantly associated with depression among the elderly respondents.

Nguyen H. and Zimmerman (2006) conducted a study reveals the relationship between the age aspects and depression. Results indicate a reasonable degree of stability among adults under 70 years of age .However there were significant age- related increases in somatic symptoms and lack of well-being after approximately 70 years of age Where as symptoms related to depressed affect the interpersonal problems and remained stable. The addition of co morbid physical illness to the analysis did not reduce the association between age and depressive symptoms.

Jakobsson U. (2006) conducted study on quality of life among older adults with arthritis (n=168) had more pain functional limitations and lower quality of life (physical\component than those without osteoarthritis (n=246) .No significant differences between the groups were found related to depressed mood and mental components of quality of life. Quality of life was associated with pain, functional limitations and depressed mood in both groups.

Radha Krishnan, (2006) assessed depression among geriatric out patients attending selected hospitals at Belgaum, Karnataka concluded that 63% of the geriatric out patients had mild to moderate depression &17% of them had severe depression according to GDs 15 and there is significant association between the level of depression and loss of spouse.

Stark Stein S. E. (2005) stated that the construct of minor and major depression among seniors in long term residential care and found that twenty six percent of the patients had major depression ,twenty six percent had mild depression and 48 percent were not depressed.

Wilson K (2006) conducted a study reveals that a prevalence rate of 21 percent and an annual incidence of 12.8 percent (Geriatric depression score of five or more) were found Risk factors associated with prevalence depression include not living close to friends and family ,poor satisfaction with living accommodation and poor satisfaction with finances. Subsequent development of clinically significant depressive symptoms was associated with base line increased scores in depression.

Sherina M. S et. al., (2006) the prevalence of depression among elderly in a tertiary care centres in Wilayah Persekutan. The results showed that 54 percent of the elderly respondents were found to have depressive symptoms age, sex, ethnicity, functional disabilities in bathing, grooming, dressing, using the toilet, transferring from bed to chair and back, mobility and climbing chairs were all found to be significantly associated with depression among the elderly respondents.

Nguyen H. and Zimmerman (2006) conducted a study reveals the relationship between the age aspects and depression. Results indicate a reasonable degree of stability among adults under 70 years of age .However there were significant age- related increases in somatic symptoms and lack of well-being after approximately 70 years of age Where as symptoms related to depressed affect the interpersonal problems and remained stable. The addition of co morbid physical illness to the analysis did not reduce the association between age and depressive symptoms.

Jakobsson U. (2006) conducted study on quality of life among older adults with arthritis (n=168) had more pain functional limitations and lower quality of life (physical\component than those without osteoarthritis (n=246) .No significant differences between the groups were found related to depressed mood and mental components of quality of life. Quality of life was associated with pain, functional limitations and depressed mood in both groups.

Radha Krishnan, (2006) assessed depression among geriatric out patients attending selected hospitals at Belgaum, Karnataka concluded that 63% of the geriatric out patients had mild to moderate depression & 17% of them had severe depression according to GDs 15 and there is significant association between the level of depression and loss of spouse.

D'Amato (2004) developed a theory of positive mental health. In his research, theories and definitions purporting to address mental health were discussed and critiqued, and a new theory of mental health was outlined. The newly developed theory accounted for neglected areas in past research regarding context and degree when defining psychological health. The new theory stated that positive mental health was reflected in the accuracy of an individual's schemata, in each of the defined schematic components, for internal and external environments.

Reddysubramaniyam G. (2005) stated that global population ageing is an important challenge and action has to be taken by virtually all countries .The geriatric population was about 600 million in 2000.It is expected to raise up to 1.2 billion in 2025 and 2 billion in 2050.About two thirds of all older persons are living in the developed countries this figure, by 2025 will be about 75%. In developing countries like India these figures have changed the nature of demands on the health care system. Health delivery system has to accommodate the needs of the older population.

White et al., (2006) conducted study on cognitive, emotional and quality of life outcomes in patients with pulmonary arterial hypertension. Results shows that cognitive sequelae occurred in 58 percent (27/46) of the pulmonary arterial hypertension patient's .Patients with cognitive sequelae had worse verbal learning delayed verbal memory, executive function, and fine motor scores compared to patients without cognitive sequelae. 26 percent of patients had moderate to severe depression and 19 percent had moderate to severe anxiety. Depression, anxiety and quality of life were not different for patients with or without sequelae. Patients had decrease quality of life, which was associated with worse working memory.

Andreoletti et. al., (2006) conducted a study on age differences in the relationship between anxiety and recall. The results shows that a negative relationship between cognitive-specific anxiety and memory, such that greater anxiety was related to poor recall, but this was so only for middle aged and older results suggest that managing anxiety may be a promising avenue for minimizing episodic memory problems in later life.

Routaslo et. al., (2006) study conducted on social contacts and their relationship to loneliness among aged people results declares that more than one third of the respondents39.4suffered from loneliness. Feeling of loneliness was not associated with the frequency of contacts with children and friends but rather with expectations and satisfaction of these contacts. The most powerful predictors of loneliness were living alone, depression, experienced poor understanding by the nearest and unfulfilled expectations of contacts with friends.

Archana singh et.al. (2009) study was conducted to investigate the relationships among depression, loneliness and sociability in elderly people. This study was carried out on 55 elderly people (both men and women). The tools used were Beck Depression Inventory, UCLA Loneliness Scale and Sociability Scale by Eysenck. Results revealed a significant relationship between depression and loneliness

Bjørkløf G.H 2013 examine Seventy-five studies, 38 clinical and 37 community settings, were included. Of these, 44 were evaluated to be of higher quality. Studies recruiting samples of older persons with a major depressive disorder, moderate or severe cognitive impairment or those who were dependent on care were scarce, thus the research is not representative of such samples. We found a huge variety of instruments assessing resources and strategies of coping (55 inventories). Although we found the relation between resources and strategies of coping and depression to be strong in the majority of studies, i.e. a higher sense of control and internal locus of control, more active strategies and positive religious coping were significantly associated with fewer symptoms of depression both in longitudinal and cross-sectional studies in clinical and community settings.

CHAPTER 3

METHODOLOGY

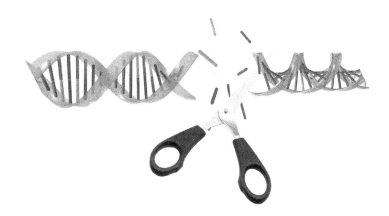

For successful study scientific methodology is necessary as it directly indicates towards the authenticity of the research. Research methodology of any research work is basic foundation through which blue print of tools and techniques are prepared to be followed during the full course of study. So method and materials appropriate for the study on **Assessment of mental health of elderly staying in old age home.** The procedure is presented order following section-

    3.1 Research design

    3.2 Locale of the study

    3.3 Sampling and sample size

    3.4 Selection of variable

    3.5 Collection of data

    3.6 Analysis and interpretation of data

3.1 Research design-

The research used for present study was descriptive in nature. Study was to know the mental health of elderly staying in old age home.

3.2 Locale of the study-

The present study is based on urban sample of 400 individual aged 60 and over. Six old age homes selected in Lucknow city selected for the data collection. **Luck**now the capital city of the Indian state of Uttar

Pradesh, was historically known as the Awadh fondly known as the _City of Nawabs' or the _City of Tehzeeb', it has always been a city filled with varied cultures. The city has been given various other names too, such as The Constantinople of India, Shiraz-i-Hind and the Golden City of the East. Lucknow has always been known as a multicultural city that flourished as a North Indian cultural and artistic hub, and the seat of power of Nawabs in the 18th and 19th centuries. Today it is the administrative headquarters of the eponymous district and Lucknow division. It is the eleventh most popular city and the twelfth most popular urban agglomeration of India. The city stands at an elevation of approximately 123 meters (404 ft) above sea level. Lucknow district covers an area of 2,528 square kilometers (976 sq mi). Bounded on the east by Barabanki, on the west by Unnao, on the south by Raebareli and in the north by Sitapur, Lucknow sits on the north-western shore of the Gomti River. It continues to be an important centre of governance, administration, education, commerce, aerospace, finance, pharmaceuticals, technology, design, culture, tourism, music and poetry. It has been listed as the 17th fastest growing city in India and 74th in the world. Lucknow, along with Agra and Varanasi, is in the Uttar Pradesh Heritage Arc, a chain of survey triangulations created by the Government of Uttar Pradesh to boost tourism in the state. Today, it is known as one of the most important cities of the country which is now emerging in various sectors like retailing, manufacturing and commercial.

The specific objectives of the study are:

1. To understand the functioning of the old age homes with regard to service provision

2. To know the mental health of elderly in old age home.

3.   To know the various health problems experienced by the elderly their management of the same.

4.   To know the opinion of the elderly regarding the adequacy of facilities and services, their satisfaction and their views on such institutional living.

5.   To identify the various problems in ensuring the smooth functioning of the old age homes.

3.3 Sampling and sample size-

Purposive random sampling was used in this study. The sample size of the study was restricted up to 400 samples. Sample selection is the important procedure to deal with the study. The data collected using a PGI battery for assessment of mental health efficiency in the elderly and observation technique through an old age home survey. The data on institutionalized was collected for most of the individuals included in the present study were 60 years of age or above. The data was collected using an especially scale design by Dr. Adarsh kohli, Dr. S.R. sharma, Dr. Dwarka Pershad department of psychology. The final data collection, the interview schedule was tested on a small sample and subsequently finalized upon successful testing. The interview schedule was divided in to five sections. The first section included question regarding general information of the respondent. The second section included question old age people memory. The third section included question standard ten test. The fourth section included sub test related to measure of perception and motion equity. The last section included questions related to depression of aging people regarding the personal interest and hobbies of old age people. P.G.I. battery of mental efficiency (MEE) is a useful tool for the aged. It is simple, easy, quick and promising tool.

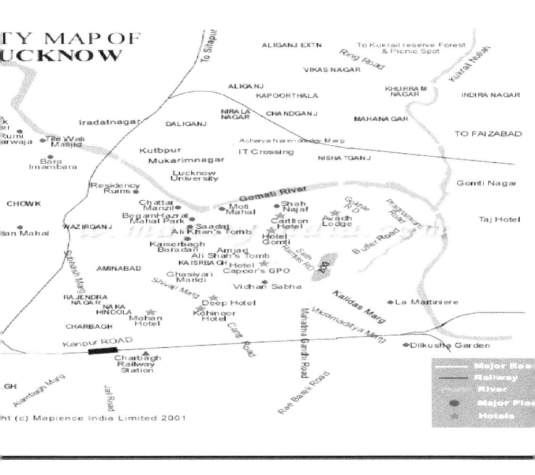

```
                            ┌──────────┐
                            │   U.P.   │
                            └────┬─────┘
                                 ↓
                            ┌──────────┐
                            │ LUCKNOW  │
                            └────┬─────┘
```

MAHANAGAR	ADIL NAGAR	JANKIPURAM	RAJAJIPURAM

ha Old Age Home	Samarpan	Chavi Shanti Dham	Sulekha Old Age Home

0	Male 50	Female 30	Male 30	Female 50	Male 50	Female 60

TOTAL 400

SAMPLE DESIGN

It takes into account the different aspects which are affected in old age, including the depression which colours their efficiency level and if moderately high can give an impression of pseudo-dementia.by giving a profile for normal as well as depressives, one can differentiate between those who are within normal range and those whose mental efficiency has really gone down. The areas measured is quite vast and comprehensive one and include memory, perceptual motor functions motivation, alertness, orientation, etc, and likely to prove useful in assessing the mental efficiency level of the elderly .

3.4 Selection of variable-

In the present study independent and dependent variable were to taken to find out the mental health between the detail about these variables and tools that were used to measure them were give is follow-

Independent variable-The independent variable is the factor that is measured manipulated or selected by observes phenomena. For the present investigation age, sex was selected independent variable.

Dependent variable: - The independent variable is factor that is measured to determine the effect of independent variable.

3.5 **Collection of data:-** The main tools used in this study a P.G.I. battery of mental efficiency (MEE) Cognitive examination scale, which consist of general and specific information required for study. ―Older people's health survey questionnaire" was used to health status of elderly people. ―Checklist for evaluating old age homes" was used to elicit data.

3.6 Analysis and interpretation of data:-

The data obtained was planned to analyze in terms of the objectives of the study using descriptive & inferential statistics. The plan of data analysis was adopted accordingly.

The collected data was coded and transformed to SPSS for statistical analysis. Demographic data was planned to represent in term of frequency and percentage.

The formula were used-

$$\text{Percentage (\%)} = \frac{\text{no. of respondent belonging to particular category}}{\text{Total no. of respondent}} \times 100$$

CHAPTER 4

RESULTS

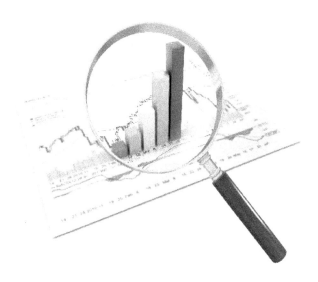

Finding of the study as obtain on the analysis of data collection by the manual for the PGI battery for assessment of mental efficiency in the elderly for systematic presentation the data. Analysis of the data collected by the older people's health survey questionnaire and checklist for evaluating old age homes are reported under following head:-

4.1- Description of sample

4.2.1-Mental health of respondents

4.2.2-Perceptual and motor activity of respondents

4.2.3-Depression of the respondents

4.3- Facilities and services of old age homes

4.4.1- Health status of respondents

4.4.2-Sensory screening and loss old people

4.4.3- Eyesight

4.4.4-Physical functioning

4.4.5- Walking aids

4.4.6-Activities of daily living

4.4.7-Psychological distress

4.4.8- Diabetes and blood sugar

4.4.9-Women health

4.4.10-Physical activity

4.1 Description of sample

This section deals with the description of the sample information pertinent to the back ground characteristics of respondents through questionnaire. The findings related to personal characteristics that are age of respondent, gender, education are presented:-

Table 4.1(1) Distribution of respondents according to age.

S.NO.	AGE GROUP	RESPONDENTS	PERCENTAGE	TOTAL
1.	60 -70 YEARS	155	39%	155
2.	71 -80 YEARS	117	29%	117
3.	81 -ABOVE	128	32%	128
TOTAL		400	100%	400

Table 4.1(1) the above table shows that 39% respondents belongs to60-70 years.29%respondents had71-80 years and 32% respondents were 81years.

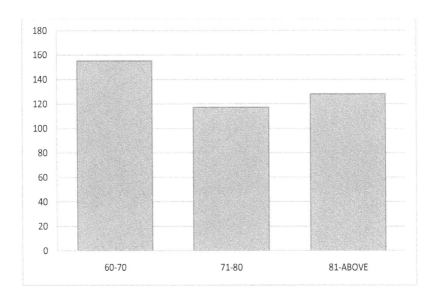

Figure 4.1(1) Graphical representation of respondents according to age.

Table 4.1 (2) Distribution of respondents on the basis of gender.

S.NO.	RESPONDENT	FREQUENCY	PERCENTAGE	TOTAL
1.	MALE	115	29%	115
2.	FEMALE	285	71%	285
	TOTAL=	400	100%	400

Table 4.1(2) the above table shows that 29% were male respondents and 71% Female respondents.

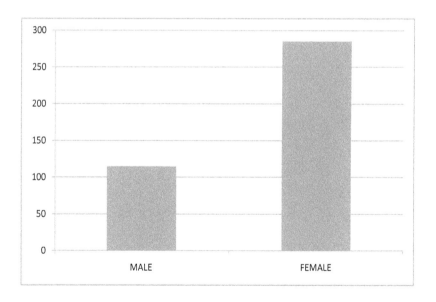

Figure 4.1(2) Graphical representation of respondents according to gender.

Table 4.1(3) Distribution of respondents according to education level

S.NO.	EDUCATION	FREQUENCY	PERCENTAGE	TOTAL=
1.	ILLETRATE	75	18%	75
2.	HIGH SCHOOL	114	28%	114
3.	INTERMEDIATE	43	10%	43
4.	UNDER GRADUTE	101	25%	101
5.	POST GRADUTE	67	16%	67
TOTAL=		400	100%	400

The data in table 4.1(3) showed that 18% respondent belongs to illiterate category.28% respondent high school education level.10% respondent intermediate and 25% belong to under graduate level. Only 6% respondent had post graduate level.

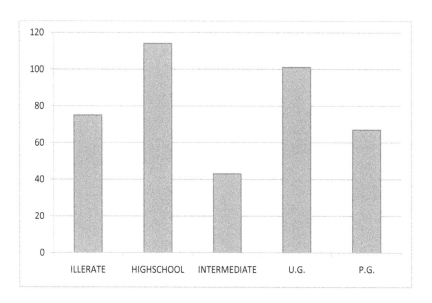

Figure 4.1(3) Graphical representation according to education level

Table 4.2(1) Distribution of respondent according to score obtain on mental health.

S.NO.	CATEGORY	FREQUENCY	PERCENTAGE	TOTAL
1.	MILD	10	2%	10
2.	MODERATE	60	15%	60
3.	SEVERE	330	83%	330
TOTAL=		400	100%	400

Table showed that distribution of respondent on the score obtain according to mental health result showed the 2%respondent had mild category. Most of the respondent82% were severe category.15% respondent belong to moderate category

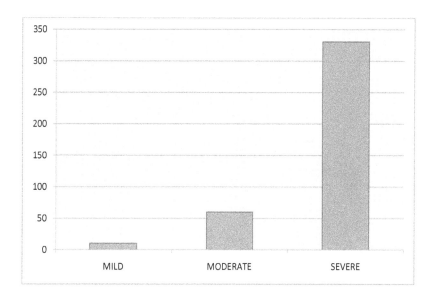

Figure4.3 Graphical representation of respondents mental health.

Table 4.2.2 Distribution of respondents according to measure of perception and motor activity.

S.NO.	CATEGORY	FREQUENCY	PERCENTAGE	TOTAL=
1.	HIGHER	172	43%	172
2.	LOWER	228	57%	228
TOTAL=		400	100%	400

Table 4.2(2) showed the distribution of respondents on the score obtain according to measure of perception and motor activity category. Result showed that 43% respondents were higher category and 57% belongs to lower category.

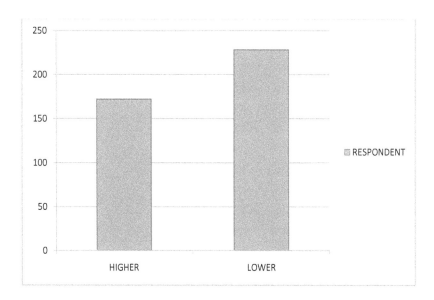

Figure 4.2(2) Graphical representation of respondent according to measure of perception and motor activity.

Table 4.2.3 Distribution of respondent according to depression scale.

S.NO.	CATEGORY	FREQUENCY	PERCENTAGE	TOTAL
1.	NORMAL	28	7%	28
2.	MODERATE	260	65%	260
3.	SEVERE	112	28%	112
TOTAL=		400	100%	400

Table 4.2(3) showed the distribution of respondent on the score obtain according to depression category. Result showed that 7%respondent were normal category. Most of the respondent 65% belong to moderate category and 28% respondent had severe category.

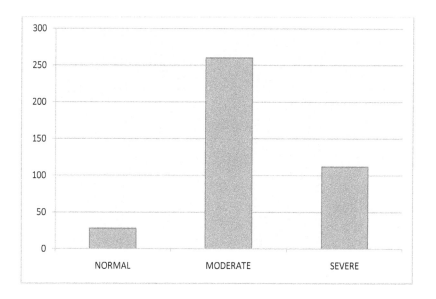

Figure 4.2(3) Graphical representation according depression level

TABLE 4.3 Distribution of respondents according to facilities and services of old home.

	SERVICE AND FACILITIES OF OLD AGE HOME	F	%
1	Do you have business registration certificate?		
	Yes	373	93
	No	27	7
2.	Lift available for access by the resident?		
	Yes	179	45
	No	221	55
3.	Are the meals adequate in amount and variety?		
	Yes	188	47
	No	211	53
4.	Does the menu offer choice for residents with special needs, such as thosewith diabetes, vegetarian on swallowing difficulty?		
	Yes	263	66
	No	137	34
TOTAL		400	100

Table 4.3(1) showed the distribution of respondents on the score obtain according to facilities and services. 93% respondents had registration certificate. Only 7% respondents had not registration certificate. Majority of respondents (55%) had home is not located at ground floor. Lift was available to the residents.45% respondents do not lift available for access by the residents. 47% respondents had simple exercise equipment and recreational facilities and 53% respondents had not simple exercise equipment and recreational facilities. 68%

respondents had meals adequate in amount and variety. Only 31% respondents had not adequate amount and Variety. 66% respondents had menu offer choices for residents with special needs such as those with diabetes vegetarian or swallowing difficulty and only 34% respondents were menu offer choices for residents with special needs.

Table4.4 (1)Health status of old people

Health status	No.(n=400)	Percentage
Excellent	10	2
Very good	50	12
Good	40	10
Fair	80	20
poor	220	55
Health problem		
yes	280	70
No	120	30
Total	400	100

Table 4.4.1 result in the table showed that about 55% respondents that they are poor health status.20%respondents had fair health status.10%respondents were good health status. most of the respondents 70% had health problems that cause difficulty in getting around and doing things for them self.30% respondents were not health problem that cause difficulty in getting around and doing things for them self.

Table4.4 (2)Sensory screening and loss old people

Sensory and screening	No.(n=400)	percentage
Hearing test		
yes	266	67
no	134	33
Use hearing aids		
Yes	186	46
no	214	54
Hearing		
excellent	10	2
good	38	9
Fair	106	26
poor	246	63
Total	400	100

Table 4.4(2) result in the table showed that majority of respondents 67% had hearing tested and 33%repondents did not checked hearing tested.46% respondents were currently use hearing aids and 56%respondents had not used hearing aids.2% elderly had excellent hearing,9%respondentsgood hearing and 26% respondents fair hearing most of the respondents 63%were poor hearing level.

Table4.4(3)Eyesight

Eyesight	No.(n=400)	Percentage
Eyesight checked		
yes	390	97
No	10	3
Wear glass for reading	243	61
For distance vision	98	24
No glass	59	15
Long distance eyesight		
Excellent	10	2
good	25	7
fair	127	32
Poor	238	59
Total	400	100

Table 4.4(3) results showed that most of respondents97% had eye sight checked; only 3% respondents were not eyesight checked. Most of the respondents(61%) had wear glass for reading and 24% were respondents wear glass for distance vision. Only 15% respondents not used glasses.2% respondents had excellent long distance eyeshight.7% respondents were good long distance eyesight.32% respondent had fair long distance eye sight. Most of the respondents had poor long distance eyesight.

Table4.4 (4)Physical functioning

Health limit you in doing vigorous activities	No.(n=400)	Percentage
Yes	372	93
No	28	7
Health limit bathing or dressing		
Yes	38	10
No	362	90
Total	400	100

Table 4.4(4) revealed that 93% respondents had health limit in doing vigorous activities.7% respondents were not health limit in doing vigorous activities.10% respondents had health limit bathing or dressing and 90% respondents were not health limit bathing or dressing.

Table 4.4(5)Walking aids

Do you currently use	No.(n=400)	percentage
A cane or walking stick	59	15
A walker farm	31	8
A wheel chair	21	5
Don"t use any aids	289	72
Total	400	100

Table 4.4(5) revealed that15% respondents had used a cane or walking stick.8% respondents used a walker frame. Very few 5% respondents had used wheel chair and most of the respondents not used any aids.

Table 4.4(6)Activities of daily living

Household duties like laundry or dusting your own	No.(n=400)	Percentage
Yes	117	29
No	283	71
Maintain gardening on your own		
Yes	19	5
No	381	95
Need help or supervision with personal care		
Yes	379	94
No	21	6
Need help cutting your toenails		
Yes	279	70
No	121	30
Total	400	100

Table 4.4(6) the above table showed that 29% respondent had household duties like laundry, vacuuming, or dusting on your own. Most of the respondents 71 % were not perform household duties like laundry, vacuuming, or dusting on your own. Only 5% respondents home maintain or gardening task on your own. most of the respondents95% were not home maintain or gardening task on your own.94% respondents had need help or supervision with personal care such as showering or bathing dressing, or getting to the toilet.6% respondents did not need help or

supervision with personal care such as showering or bathing dressing, or getting to the toilet. Most of the respondents70% had need help cutting their toenails.30% respondents were not need help cutting their toenails.

Table 4.4(7)Psychological distress

Feel so sad that nothing could cheer you up	No.(n=400)	Percentage
All of the time	47	12
Most of the time	188	47
Some of the time	97	24
A little of the time	68	17
Total	400	100

Table 4.4(7) Result in the table showed that 12%respondents feel so sad that nothing cheer them. Majority 47% respondents had most of time feel so sad that nothing cheer them .24% respondents some of the time feel so sad that nothing could cheer them. Only 17% respondents feel so sad that nothing could cheer them.

Table 4.4(8)Diabetes and high blood sugar

Have diabetes	No=(n=400)	Percentage
Yes	287	72
No	113	28
Total	400	100

Table 4.4(8) revealed that 72% respondent had diabetes and high blood sugar and 28%respondents were not diabetes and high blood sugar.

Table 4.4(9)Women health (for women only)

Had a mammogram	No.(n=230)	percentage
Yes	46	20
No	184	80
Did you last have a mammogram less than 1 year ago	15	7
5 or more years age	31	13
Never	184	80
Clinical breast examination		
Yes	97	42
No	133	58
Total	230	100

Table 4.4(9) result in the table showed that 20% respondents had meomgramme and 80% respondents were not memogramme.7% respondents had a memogramme 1 year ago to less then 2 years ago and 13% respondents

Table 4.4(10) Physical activity

Physical active compare to others	No.(n=400)	Percentage
Much less active	89	22
About as active	98	24
A bit more active	79	20
Much more active	134	33

Table 4.4(10) result in the table showed that 22% respondents physically active compare to other. Majority33% of respondents had more active. Only 20% respondents not more active compare to others.

CHAPTER 5

DISCUSSION

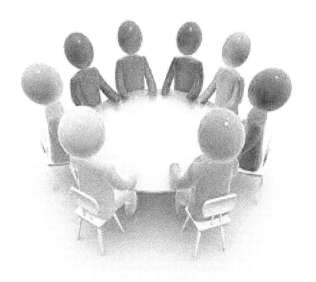

A total of 7 old age homes were found to functional to Lucknow. Five to them were selected to get and overview of facilities and services of old age homes. All of these old age homes were residential and having the provision to accommodate both male and female older adults. Majority of the inhabitants of these old age homes were between the age group of 60 to 81 above. The reason could be significantly more psychological stress, lack of family support, lack of medical facilities, restricted environment of old age homes, further similar studies are needed to evaluate finding the study. This study was conducted for evaluating mental health of elderly staying in old age homes of Lucknow city. The analysis of mental health and various health problems of aged people enable the researcher to understand nature, extent of various problem faced by them. It is better to present consolidated picture of the study.

The main findings of the survey are as follows-

❖ There are two types of old age homes. One is the government organization which facility is _free' types which cares for the destitute who have no one else to care of they are given shelter, food clothing and medical care. The second type is the nongovernment organization where care is provided for a fee.

❖ Old age home are located in a pleasant quiet atmosphere. It is some open ground so that the old can move about freely and safely for exercise relaxation or peace of mind. Recreation room available. This creates pleasant atmospheres around the old age homes. All old age homes have sufficient facilities. They were happy about the facilities provided to them.

❖ Nongovernment organization given best facilities and services compare to government organization.

❖ General information about respondents age wise distribution was as follows 39% respondents belongs to60-70years.29%respondents had71-80 years and 32%respondents were 81above years.29% were male respondents and 71% female respondents. 18% respondents belong to illiterate category. Majority (28%) respondent's high school education level.10% respondents intermediate and 25% belong to under graduate level. Only 6% respondents had post graduate level.

❖ As regards the depression problem of the elderly people. It was found that 65% of respondents feel moderate category of depression in the old age homes. This is because many of them do not maintain their family contact and they are suffering from some sort of physical ailments.

❖ In the study, it was found that all the respondents face some mental health problems. Table4.3 shows the82% of the respondents belongs to severe category of depression.

❖ Respondents on the score obtain according to measure of perception and motor activity category. Result showed that 43% respondents were higher category and 57% belongs to lower category.

❖ Respondents on the score obtain according to facilities and services 93% respondents had home display the business registration certificate. Only 7% respondents were home display the business registration certificate. Majority of respondents 55% had home is not located at ground floor is lift available for access by the residents.45% respondents do not lift available for access by the residents. 47% respondents had simple exercise equipment and recreational facilities and 53% respondents do not simple exercise equipment and recreational facilities. 68% respondents had meals adequate in amount and variety and only 31% respondents belong to meals adequate amount and Varity. 66% respondents had menu offer choices for residents with special needs such as those with diabetes vegetarian or swallowing difficulty and only 34% respondents were menu offer choices for residents with special needs.

❖ Most of the respondents 70% had health problems that cause difficulty in getting around and doing things for your self. 30% respondents were not health problem that cause difficulty in getting around and doing things for your self. result in the table showed that majority of respondents 67% had hearing tested and 33%repondents did not checked hearing tested.46% respondents were currently use hearing aids and 56%respondents had not used hearing aids.2% elderly had excellent hearing,9%respondentsgood hearing and 26% respondents fair hearing most of the respondents 63%were poor hearing level.

❖ Most of respondent (97%) had eye sight checked, only 3% respondents were not eyesight checked. It was also found that most of the respondents had poor long distance eyesight Only 2% respondents had excellent long distance eye sight.

❖ Very few 10% respondents had health limit bathing or dressing and most of them 90% respondents were not health limit bathing or dressing.

❖ Most of the respondents do not used any aids very few 5% respondents had used wheel chair.

❖ Only 5% respondents home maintain or gardening task on your own. 94% respondents had need help or supervision with personal care such as showering or bathing dressing, or getting to the toilet. In which 70% had need help cutting your toenails.

❖ Result in the table showed that 12%respondents feel so sad that nothing could cheer you up.47% respondents had most of time feel so sad that nothing could cheer up.24%respondents were some of the time feel so sad that nothing could cheer you up. Only 17% respondents a little of the time feel so sad that nothing could cheer you up.

❖ It was found that 72% respondent had diabetes and high blood sugar and 28%respondents were not diabetes and high blood sugar.

❖ Table 4.4.9 result in the table showed that 20% respondents have you ever had meomgramme and majority 80% respondents were not had a memogramme.7% respondents had a memogramme 1 year ago to less then 2 years ago and 13% respondents.

❖ All the respondents have reported that they are fully satisfied and do not have any problem in the institution. They gain a feeling of security and compassion from other inmates who belong to the similar age group, having similar attitude and interest .Besides personal care is offered to them by the staff in these institutions.

❖   All the respondents are of the view that institutional life can be substitute for family life, nevertheless it can be concluded that in the present society old age home offer great relief for the aged. In this study the researcher tried his best to elicit the problem of the elderly and welfare measures taken by old age homes.

CHAPTER 6

SUMMARY AND CONCLUSION

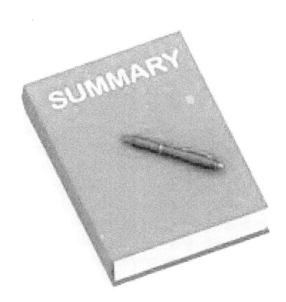

This study examined the assessment of mental health of elderly staying in old age homes of old age homes in Lucknow city is the result of a study conducted by the researcher using detailed literature review, personal interviews and statistical techniques. The researcher followed computerized analysis. SPSS is used for analyzing the data. Tables and graphs were used in analysis, adequate interpretation was drawn out regarding variables.Nongovernment organization given best facilities and services provide to compare government organization. An older person with mental health problem experiences many forms of discrimination as a result; their view and experiences remain largely invisible policy practices and research. This limits both range and quality of services and support that are available to them and lead to in equalities both within the older population and between different age.

❖ Older people who experience mental health problems and need of their cares are understood taken seriously given their fair share of attention and resources.

❖ Older people's mental health services have been systematically disadvantage, suffering from low level of investment, low priority on multiple agendas and low individual expectation of mental health in later life.

❖ The prevalence of mental health problem as well as physical problem was found to be higher in inhabitants of old age homes.

❖ The increase in the number of older people is inevitable and welcome and we must insure that the number of older people who suffer mental health problems are minimised. We have the opportunity and the knowledge to make changes that will help our society and our economy and prevent enormous suffering in the future. We must accept the challenge and take action now.

❖ Depression was found to be most common mental disorder. Dementia and schizophrenia in male and anxiety and dementia in female support earlier finding.

❖ Older people with mental health problems who are not using services at least half of older people with mental health problems like depression and dementia are never diagnosed and few ever receive treatment. These older people are likely to be relying on support from family and friends, who may also be older and in need of support themselves.

❖ It has been found that majority of respondents lived with their families, before joining the old age home but they were forced to leave their home because of various reasons problems of health, problem of family indifference, economic insecurity, problem of loneliness, psychological insecurity, conflict in status and role, problem of recreation etc.

Recommendations

❖ The government must support to the old age homes. Then they can improve their facilities.

❖ Government must look at old age people who cannot afford to pay with the pension and government subsidy.

❖ The younger generation should be made aware of the love and care needed by the old people.

❖ Research is needed on the psychology of the old aged, efficacy of services for the aged, and health and nutritional problems of the aged.

❖ Old age homes should be designed in such a way that they must physically and psychologically be conductive to the aged people.

❖ Social workers can help the elderly they should be aware about the various policies and programme related to the welfare of the aged in our country. This will help the elderly to protect their rights.

❖ There is a need to build the capacity to staff through regular training programme. This would allow staff to be updated with the most recent practices in the care of older persons.

❖ Free medical care may be provided with the help of some organizations. It is recommended that funding policies should be re-addressed as many of less affluent homes or struggling to maintain health care standards.

❖ Forming organizations of elder lies and caretakers will be a great help.

❖ To help them psychologically counselling classes can be arranged. Government should look at separate facilities to accommodate patients with Alzheimer, Dementia and mental illness. These require specialist forms of care as well as trained specialist staff required to provide optimum care.

❖ Spiritual care is necessary for the aged. Most of them tend to be deeply religious and spiritual. So pastoral care may be given to them.

CPSIA information can be obtained
at www.ICGtesting.com
Printed in the USA
BVHW071039130223
658295BV00015B/1809